TRYING TO REMEMBER

TRYING TO REMEMBER

A Family's Journey Through Alzheimer's

ANNE CROSSMAN

YELLOW WOOD PRESS

ISBN: 978-0-557-01732-4

In remembrance of Betty McClure Nicholas,
that which she has forgotten,
and that which we cannot forget

෨

In honor of Payson King Nicholas,
for fifty-three years
in sickness and in health

As for man, his days are like grass;
As a flower of the field, so he flourishes.
When the wind has passed over it, it is not more,
And its place acknowledges it no longer.

Psalms 103:15-16

CONTENTS

DIAGNOSIS

Before Teeing Off

She hasn't been herself lately. I suggested making
love. Would you believe my bride,
who fifty years ago wouldn't kiss me
until I proposed, agreed
but said I had to hurry —
her husband came home at eight?

Add-a-pearl Necklace

It was the family joke that he —
ever the accountant —
wed at year's end to claim dependants
while I was born costing money.

A New Year's baby, my arrival was a sore spot
when his wife witnessed my homecoming
instead of coming home.
Their thirty-seventh anniversary
came the day before my birth — fitting,
I've thought, since their love led to me.

Every year it was the same. For my birthday
she would give me a pearl
and a teddy bear calendar
with the note *On your happy day.*
The necklace would be restrung
and I would count my new age with my teeth,
sliding each pearl like a chorus line
across my gentle bite.

When her handwriting wasn't hers on my eighth,
I didn't notice. When my ninth turned
from Teddy to tulips I dismissed my mother's cursive
and bit down on the gritty pearl.
We never spoke of the absent
bears or altered scrawl. She would surrender the gift each year
This is from Grandma
and another pearl would be added.

The Mini Mental State Examination for Alzheimer's in Recitative

Madam, put away your pocketbook
and listen very clearly—
I want you to list off today's
exact date to the year, please.
Well done. Now, without peeking,
recall our building's name,
what floor we're on, what day
it is, and are we now in Maine?
And how about our season, this
neighborhood, our city?
I'm going to list off three things,
repeat them nice and pretty.
Ready? *candle, hammer, heart.*
Oh, do not feel encumbered.
Count backwards from one hundred
naming every seventh number.
So far so good, you're doing great,
we're nearly almost done.
Can you repeat the objects
from before, now one by one?
What is this and what is that?
You're doing fine—you're not a nut—
now echo me but do not laugh
no if's, and's, or but's.
Splendid, here's some paper.
Now hold it to your right,
fold it up, lay it flat,
and put it out of sight.
Close your eyes,
now open them and write

a sentence please.
Oh, any topic's fine
just as long as it's complete.
One more drill and then we're done,
here's a piece of paper:
draw intersecting pentagons.
Great! We'll see you later!

Did you pass and are you crazy?
Oh, please, let's not ask questions.
You did your best and that's what counts.
Let's schedule one more session.

Old-Timers

Why can't I remember?
I have Alzheimer's—
old-timers, I like to call it.
They say someday I'll forget everything.
That can't be right.

Why can't I remember?
Oh watchamacalit.
Nick, whats-it again?
You say someday I'll forget
every-you?
That's not right.

Why cand I remember?
You don't kno wit.
My time is old.
They say everything
not trite.

Hy cand I?
Cand bemmer wy.

Stage Three

I am afraid of the forgetting
that has come. I am afraid that the awkwardness
of my hollowing mind will be more than my loved
ones can bear. I am afraid of losing any decency
and the knowledge I should apologize.
I am afraid to be without memory's comfort.

I am hopeless and nothing can comfort
me when I find myself forgetting
more than I let on. I could apologize
but admitting my insanity would be awkward.
Besides, I should be aging decently,
dying with dignity for those I love.

I am worried I'll lose their respect and love
as they go poor keeping me comfortable.
What will slip from my lips indecently,
once my guard is down for good and I forget
how to bite my tongue? What infantile awkwardness
will finally drive them away after I can't apologize?

I taught my three children to apologize
quickly so that bitterness won't kill love.
If only I could confess my awkwardness
in advance — yet another comfortless
wish that cannot numb my forgetting.
My memory's nakedness takes from today's decency

and leaves me dreading which of tomorrow's decencies
will be molested without apology.
Those who don't understand think my forgetting
is a convenient excuse to erase unloved
memories and dwell on more comforting
thoughts. Telling them the awkward

truth makes the conversation doubly awkward.
No one has given me the decency
of choosing which memories to keep, no one can comfort
me that this will all be over soon, no one can apologize
for my loss — it's no one's fault my loved
ones will soon be part of what's forgotten.

My head throbs when I think of what I'll forget.
There's a lot there to lose. I remember the awkward
time I told Nick *No ring, no kiss* and worried his love
might run. I remember Mother's lessons on decency —
to always carry a clean hankie and to apologize
promptly if we disturbed Father's comfort.

I remember my children's laughter and how I would comfort
skinned-knees with a silly song to make them forget
the sting. I'm rambling and I apologize
but I have to repeat what I know to keep the awkward
growth from growing. These stories sound senseless
but even all mixed up in my mind they remind me I'm loved.

Most days my mind gets tongue tied — for the love
of pete I can't make meaning from the confusing
mess. It makes me so mad I lose all good sense
about not swearing in front of little ears who forget
much less than I do. Back-peddling awkwardly
I excuse my French and hope to whisper a bedtime apology.

Our friends don't bother anymore with excuses or apologies
about why they don't call. Of course, we'd love
to play a round with them but small talk would be awkward.
*So, Betty, gotten lost in any good alleys lately? Confused
the milkman for Nick yet?* Though they'd never say, I'm betting
they think it. I haven't completely lost my senses.

9

Demoted from retiree to nurse, Nick tries to make sense
of the worst and is sweetly apologetic
for not being patient with me sooner. He's betting
all we've saved against me on the coming rounds, loving
the labels that stage out the list of confusions.
We ignore the invisible line between home and the ward.

In fact, we don't speak much of *it* at all, warding
off the germans eating my brain with denial. I sense
their guile: take small bites, chew thirty-two times to confuse
her she's been eaten alive. But I know my head's a thought
lighter and a pebble slower than most. I love
that you shake your noggin but you're nodding inside, I bet.

Don't feel awkward. Death is decent enough to bet
against us all. Give it an hour and I sense that in my confusion
I will have forgotten the thoughtful comfort of your loving
    apology.

Aria of the Caretaker

This is where we hang our keys
so we can find them later.

This is where we hang our keys
on this brass hook
so we can find them later.

This is where we hang our keys
on this brass hook
not in that nook
so we can find them later.

This is where we hang our keys
beside the door
on this brass hook
not in that nook
so we can find them later.

This is where we hang our keys
beside the door
above the floor
on this brass hook
not in that nook
so we can find them later.

See the sticky note by the car
This is where we hang our keys
beside the door
above the floor
on this brass hook
not in that nook
so we can find them later.

See the sticky note by the car
and the cardboard arrow marking
This is where we hang our keys
beside the door
above the floor
on this brass hook
not in that nook
so we can find them later.

The motion sensing voice explains
See the sticky note by the car
and the cardboard arrow marking
This is where we hang our keys
beside the door
above the floor
on this brass hook
not in that nook
so we can find them later.

The placards in the hall detain
so motion sensors can explain
See the sticky note by the car
and the cardboard arrow marking
This is where we hang our keys
beside the door
above the floor
on this brass hook
not in that nook
so we can find them later.

The lighting on the floor denotes
where placards in the hall detain
so motion sensors can explain
See the sticky note by the car
and the cardboard arrow marking

12

This is where we hang our keys
beside the door
above the floor
on this brass hook
not in that nook
so we can find them later.

This is a clapping key remote
which beeps when flooring won't denote
in case the placards don't detain
or motion sensors can't explain
the sticky note has fallen far
and isn't cuing by the car
in tandem with the arrow marking
This was where we hung our keys
not on the hook
but in the nook
or in the door
or on the floor
beneath the fridge
lest hell freeze over
and we find them later.

A Dead Horse Makes Poor Company

I taste this memory daily, like a pill —
refilled, familiar, and addicted
to the bitter coating.

Forgive and forget might have spared me
had I known what He meant earlier,
but the grudge
like a wedge in a wound
infects for infinity —
or at least for the length of my days.

My cabinet of recollections is rotting
but this file lies dog-eared on my desk.
Forgetting is impossible;
forgiving, a pleasantry.

Rather than alphabetize the blame
I must choose to not remember.
Easier said than stifled.

The Match

I.
Exhumed from packed snapshots
is an ashen portrait of a wizened woman seated center
in a rocker, babe in christening lace on her lap,
proud parents framing her within arms reach,
and a determined smile beneath her piled hair and weary eyes.
Scrawled on the back in pencil:
three generations.

II.
Sifting through the chest
Dress-up Mama's Darling
silken gloves match streaming gown, starring: Barbara Ann.
Clomping across her stage and runway,
the mantle's glow her limelight,
Keep away from the running flame!
embers catch the hem making molten of crinoline.
Scream-streaking through the room and I—Caretaker Doom—
could not strip her fire, cannot hush her cries,
Bury Mama's Baby
empty the chest.

III.
My body, which they said was dead and would never deliver,
did. Named for the one we no longer named,
your first breath was my pardon,
her summon, your burden: Barbara Ann.

Above the Unraveling

Everything was the color of coffee-stained teeth
—towels, commode, tile, sink, tub—

relics from an age of interior decorating
I'm glad I missed. Wafts of aqua net,

listerine, yesterday's prunes, and stale perfume clung
like the bar by their old-people's potty.

Above the unraveling where we wiped our all-clean hands
—*Betty and The Beast* or was it *Beauty and Nick*?—

order wooed humor with blue dymo-marker tape
so she'd know which towel was hers.

Belaboring Dead Horses

Mother had often said that I was crazy
to marry a man who'd been called to war,
leave my sister playing alone,
and dream of going to nursing school.
She said naming me after Father's favorite
dog made me hang off balance.

In those days we married for social balance
but nursing honeymoon babies made our husbands as crazy
as pound dogs, since they were no longer our favorites.
After a few drinks at the bar some would come home to a war
zone while others didn't, leaving with old school
chums to visit whores or their mothers, or just wandering alone.

Nursing was a world left well enough alone
by men. After the war the number of suitors was imbalanced
and mothers were forced to send daughters to school.
Well, it was that or be left old-maid crazy.
Fate had gambled with the dog tags of our men at war,
and won the one I married. He was her favorite.

After the honeymoon I was nobody's favorite.
Three days after our wedding I was left alone
when Nick shipped off to Guadal Canal, merry to fight the
    world's war.
Dogs mate for longer, Mama said, trying to balance
her worry with every other mother and wife. We were crazy
to risk widowhood when we should have gone to nursing
    school.

Had Barbara Ann lived they might have let me leave for school
instead of being dogged by grief and penance. Their favorite
baby girl we'd all nursed and coddled and loved was gone. Crazy.
Mama went crazy. We all did. Her darling had been left alone
with a fool. A fool who'd married her to Death. The balance
of our home was in forever aftershocks. Like we'd lost the war.

Only the dog will lick my war
wounds. Because I let her die, motherhood schooled
me on loss after loss after loss. My hopes for balance,
for pleasure as a newly married lover, for their favor
or at least forgiveness, and my someday nursery all died too. I
    was alone
for all those years, leaving Mother right and me crazy.

Crazed from grief because I'd left the room, and nursing a war-
torn love, worry smothered and married me unhappily ever
    after to schools
of disquiet. Not even my favorite dog can tend to my imbalance.

Stage Five

Eight times you asked your daughter,
Why's the chandelier in that tree?
She showed you the reflection
and explained it patiently.
Finally on the ninth time
she said without a grin,
That's the way it's done now
and you forgot to ask again.

Beautiful lady, who taught me cat's cradle
and signed the epilogue of my childhood,
is this another of your tricks? Like the Halloween
you drove for five hours, dressed as a masked flapper,
just to knock on our door and beg for treats?

On the slab beside our house
Grandpa camped your motor-home,
with a freezer so convenient
we bought extra waffle cones.
Once the sentinel of snack time
now you scrapped the bucket thinner
and served dessert at every whim,
forgetting room for dinner.

Last night I watched home movies and found you
unlost and remembering, tasting root beer again
like it was the first time, your once again self.
Funny how some magnets bring you back
and others expose how far you've gone.

An Independence Party,
bringing family from afar,
had you wandering past the faces
blaming that they stole your car.
Then weaving through the playroom
you spied grandkids Passing Go
and asked your hovering daughters
Are these children that I know?
As you swiveled to escape
you tripped our puppy from behind
and apologized with petting,
Smoke, I'm sorry, I've lost my mind.

Because He Could No Longer Afford to Buy Gifts

It hangs around my neck
like an heirloom millstone —
one she doesn't remember bequeathing
and wouldn't. The family agreed,
post her garbaged disposal
of an amethyst ring, pearl
brooch and sapphire pin,
to relieve her of the valuables
she could no longer value.
And so I inherited this mystery, this
piece of her memory
which she cannot remember —
just like my name
and that of her child, my mother —
but recognizes, then asks for it back.

Waltz

He doesn't come for her reaction; he comes because he loves her.

Day-shift nurse

Drawn to her easy grace,
stubbornness, simple face,
asked her to be his wife
to love and lead for life.
No time to sew a dress,
book a church, host a dance.
If he returns at all
he'll rent the biggest hall, vowing
Come with me, you will see how love can be led beautifully.

Whisking past trikes and toys
he'd woo her from their boys,
offer a steady arm,
wink, then unfold his charm.
They'd sway past laundry piles,
kitchen sink, bashful smiles,
promenade through the house,
PK and his sweet mouse, singing
Come with me, you will see how love can be led beautifully.

Time cut in on their dance,
memories gone in advance,
he chasséd by her side,
she took the twirls in stride.
New Year's Eve: celebrate
gold anniversary date.
He led her on the floor,
she followed, steps assured, humming
Come with me, you will see how love can be led beautifully.

Speechlessly she would stare,
spotting what wasn't there,
feet pitched with broken sway,
infantile, locked away.
Stereo under arm,
reintroduced with charm,
he'd ask her for a dance,
soften her empty glance, lulling
Come with me, you will see how love can be led beautifully,
as we slow I'll hold you tight, do not fear the dark of night,
next to me you'll find rest, lean your cheek against my chest,
here for you, held in true as long as breath remains in me

Caregiver Support Group: First Meeting This Thursday

Betty and I are doing fine
now that I sold our home
and divested everything for Medicare.
I nursed her as long as I could. But that day
she used Mr. Clean for cooking oil
I knew I needed help. She had become this
oversized toddler who couldn't retain why
electric curlers, parking brakes, and garbage disposals were
    dangerous.
The day she wandered for hours in alleys downtown
I knew our life was lost.
I explained our move to Rosewood
which she understood then forgot
along with my name.

I don't golf like I used to. Honestly
I'm at Betty's center so much
I don't have time. I walk two miles a day to stay in shape
since my old foursome found a fourth easily.

They don't ask how she is
not that it's important but I thought
they would. I've known Sye since Guadal Canal
and Howard from before we had children.
Their wives used to borrow Betty's mink stole.
Maybe they don't know
what to say. Or my pretending I'm fine
leaves me nothing to tell.

And that's my story. You can call me Nick
or PK. My friends call me PK.
Betty liked to call me Nick
and Payson when she was angry.

Conundrum

I've come to say goodbye to you
but don't know how to start.
It's not as though I'm leaving
or that you are wandering far.

In fact, you'll be here all the while
in body and some mind,
except that you'll be slipping, slowly
running out of time.

Should we trade our last goodbyes
while you still know my name,
so we can reminisce on kinder times
before *it* came?

Or is it wrong to rush your death
recalling what we've known,
seeming to demean your feelings,
serving just my own?

And if I wait to say so long
for when it's truly time,
what if you're already gone
and we don't say goodbye?

THE WARD

Photo Caption: Betty recites the entire 23rd Psalm

The Lord is my shepherd
and who are you, I want to know.
He makes me lie down in amber waves of grain.
He leads me beside myself.
He restakes my soul though my mind won't follow
in paths of right choices, for pete's sake.
Yea though I wander through alleys of shadows, I fear
I only know Thee.
The staff comfort me
and mash pears at the table before me
with presents for my memories.
My head needs ointment
and my cup drips.
Surely something follows all my days indivisible
I don't know what ever for.

During the War

Every day
ever ree day ea
very dea ev vree
deo effrie D
yay vary day
F-ree deuv ray
damn ef reed
dever vay red
day

I wrote him for three years.

sedatives & restraints

the current undertoes me
coma-conscious. deeper. steeper. reaper-grim. waving
sweeps of peaks,
a woe of life, a blithy moat. floating
like a boat tip-toteting the tide
whose wide-washed wearms bathe
the beauty bleaming. deep sleep keeps salt
from my eyes. then BLANDAMSLAM in my ears nose
    ohse
and there.
deep there. bitty-bits stick on pink-stubbed rub. cut
the rope. dole the dope. axons away.

Pink

My ice cream
    Frozen bits of gum
    staining lips, tongue, teeth.
    Grandpa's treat.

Its parlor
    Hosable vinyl
    squeaks when seated.
    Feeble friendly.

Our badges
    Blinding neon
    proves us The Sane Ones.
    Clip and pat often.

Her sweatshirt
    Permanent AVNC
    marked on the collar.
    Inmate for life.

His pallor
    Her hand in his pocket
    groping— *Betty, stop*
    looking for my keys.

The Real Question

Well how would you feel if after fifty years
I stared at you blankly and introduced
myself?

Would you dress me and still adore me?

What if a lifetime of travel, the birth of our
children, our romantic courtship
vanished,

Would you mutter my name as a curse?

nothing but a cavernous warehouse,
stained concrete where shelves once stood?

Would you keep record of my offences?

Sure, you could flip through old scrapbooks
and with much effort convince me I am
your wife,

Would you empty my diaper and wipe me?

but when I approach you minutes later
with pursed lips and hollow eyes,

Would you repeat sweet nothings in my ear?
Would you forget who I was?

would you begin again?

Nurses Thought We Should Know

Bobby, no
not that game
all alone
didn't stop
tried the lock
no one will
ever know
Mousie won't
tell, I fell
Nick help it
hurts, I'm lost
yes him too
he did I
mean didn't
our secret
please Daddy
don't go
my fault shows
Bobby, no

Sunday Visits with Grandma

Well I'll tell you, Honey,
tum-ton money come pell
and she tried to lie-hide him
ever dintrim in never mind
when Mother found how
pout keshtoper had funny rum
the secret was out.
Does ice cream taste you?
Dum dee-dum dee-dum dee sky true blue
and now you diddlie-dum know.

Riding Dead Horses

Dr. Shivorsenstein scours his notes,
It appears that she suffered from notable strokes
of trauma *clearing his throat to continue*
the kind that we find in molestation. Do you
know if that's the case? *We brace ourselves,*
we nod, he explains. We delve
into our patients' pasts because it seems the memories which
 last
are often those which are painful, latching
themselves deep in the brain. It's a strain to prove
but it behooves us to note that our folks loop
through traumas. Mrs. Daley, there, scares us all
when she routinely screams at a husband who beat her, the hall
nurses grieve and no one can treat or distract
'til she's done. Mr. Black, here, watches a tractor
crush Willie. Even with pills he remembers the name
and the gore. Blame keeps score and the bloody remains
of lives are on parade, often
distilled down to guilt. A coffin
may be their only escape unless therapy saves
with forgiveness. My wish is this theory could brave
the lab instead of raising hackles:
had patients knocked off their shackles
before, they might not have been scarred and perhaps
might not even be here. Shame amputates its captives
and — I'm sorry — I've lapsed
into lecture. If you have any questions — *we don't, we shake, we*
 escape,
clutching our collars where they gape.

It's Only Money

Damn. It's gone again.

How many times
before they lock me up with Mother?

I swear,
if my head wasn't attached
my shoulders would make a nice serving

Fate?
Nah,
can't be.

Gotta find that
Whatever

Was I saying something?

Now I really sound like her.

I'm on my fifth trip upstairs
and I can't remember what
I'm looking for.

This bookend of a brain is as sharp as my goldfish.

I'm amazed I remember to breathe.

Every time I go shopping
I forget the list
which does me no good on the fridge and
hey —

What's my purse doing in there?

My noggin has the pep of a chicken with freezer burn.

On a fast track to cold sheets at

The more I explain the sillier I sound.
Can't handle light conversation

or parking the car
there's a mini-van with license plate A-N-1-7-9-2...
My battery's dead in the head
and nobody's home to help.

I'm having an Alzheimer's moment.

Out to lunch
and lost my lunchbox.

The sharpest knife
and a stitch in time
still won't help my elevator.

I wonder what I'll forget first

or have
already forgotten
and don't yet

No.
Somebody shoot me
before

I forget
to do it myself.

Unscrambling Her Forgetting

Hi adee! Se Zar's slime?
E dam his lease risez!
Dame hears lies size,
seiz heal adressi me.
Side ahlariez seems
hard, miss ezie alees.
Dear, seas Leihi mesz.
Rez, heal mi diseesas.
Hearz lies me's ideas.

In the Hole

Pitter patter putter
Drive for show he would remind,
send it flying with a flutter
Put for dough a note behind.

But his motto bit the pit
one day and shuddered in the sand
when he drove with show on one grand hit
and dropped it on demand.

For forty years he swung the club
with measured skill and poise,
and on that day his hole-in-one
won drinks from all the boys.

To knock it far and fair
and see it arc from green to gulp
caused a man of the most somber air
to dance the tee to pulp.

And so, we said, what greater site
to edify his rest
than the hole that brightened up his life —
the victory he loved best.

We prodded proper channels
and we made appealing calls
but the Club preferred our mantle
to their fairway waterfall.

Displeased that they denied his
peaceful rest beside the course,
we schemed and all decided
we would claim the Third by force.

Lingering one evening
when the Club was serving drinks,
we ambled calmly on the green
to walk him to the links.

It seemed a charming stroll,
or so the gazers must have thought—
a family stopping on the knoll
to pass a copper pot.

The willow tree was neatly trimmed,
cicadas hid our prayers
as we slipped him in beneath the brim
with not an ash to spare.

Onlookers lulled our laughter
as we galloped home in measure
trying hard to hide our rafter
scaling, roof impaling pleasure.

We wink to them each round,
wave a club, and tip our caps—
then play the Third without a sound
while two share saintly naps.

Stage Seven

As I enter the foyer I make a game of the decorator's age —
fleur-de-lis upholstery, watercolor landscapes, puckered
gauze lampshades: all mauve — sixty-two.
Clicking a fluorescent Visitor (also pink) to my lapel,
the nurse compliments Mother's gentleness
before buzzing me in. It's been six months

here where there are no sedatives or restraints
just an oversized playpen.
Dad was right to move her. After a few laps I find her
napping in someone else's bed, nuzzling
a rag doll. At least she's wearing her own clothes.

With lunch on the way I take her to the lounge,
wishing for warm laundry to fold so we could talk like before.
Smoothing her hands, I search her blank blue eyes.
I try to hold her gaze
but like a pair of magnets that have tripped, we can't connect.

I tell her about her grandchildren — that three start jobs in July,
two graduate from college, and one is a bride — still folding
her hands between mine. Breaking from her vacant expression
and my threatening tears, I rise to knead piles of knots from her
     shoulders.

I don't know if she knows I'm near but I'm here just the same.
David comes three times a week
like Dad before he died and hides where I stand now: mute,
only rubbing. His voice makes her cry.
Lunch is late.

I hand her my purse like she would
when we were children, numb in a pew
by an eternal sermon, and then a glint—
fool's gold or the real McClure? She sees me

then returns to the curtains. I've lost her again.
The pinks drain to gray. I hug her
and whisper the goodbye she's never heard
though I tell her every visit. I kiss her cheek.
My tears mark her face, and as I walk away she groans.

ESCAPE

Condolences

It will all be over soon she will be out of pain full of bile her body has come to its end of her suffering a few more days perhaps she is slipping and doesn't look so good fell won't eat had an episode waiting for her passing the time has come sooner than we thought later than we hoped to think of what to say if she is leaving us for good for her.

Love Letters

Where?
Burned.
Burned?
Safe.
Lost!
Protected
Destroyed.
Proper.
Baloney.
Privacy.
Legacy.
Respect.
Neglect.
Gone.
Ef-airy one?
Yes.

End Stage

Lightness pinks my pastel and I wait for warm.
Sweet in my bones, soft on my skin,
tasty fills me with yum and someone loves me.
The new is never old and can't be
though I sing it over and over.
Today I watched a rose. A rose without foes
tickles my nose. Rest comes if weary and wake when ready
and I wonder if it's always been this good.

Looking After Grandma

I have been writing about
you since I was nine. It was
the day you didn't cry when
you forgot my name that sent
me home thinking I'd fall head
first into the heaving sky.

I used to have to work
from dark to dark and
didyouknow whose film
was on display each time
I rode the train tracks
on the crack of dawn?

Remember the time you came
to the table, bra outside
of your blouse? Imagine me
unable to say the word
bra without turning red and
in walks Grandma on display.
You were a good sport when Aunt
Barb escorted you to change.

Before I met him I worked
the theater reels and rode
the train and didn't get home
til late to feed and bathe them.

Sometimes when the wind blows warm
I feel your wrinkled kisses
whisker behind my ear where
you used to find them hiding.
When I look at my mother,
your daughter, I see you — like

a moving photograph where
part of you is alive in
someone else's laugh — and I
want them to see you in mine.

Peter Peter pumpkin eater had
a wife and da-dum keep
her da-dum-da a pumpkin
shell and there he kept her
da-da-da.

I haven't cried for you in
a while. I'm sorry for that.
A lot of me has grown up
since you left, but the part that
misses you is still waiting,
the one who couldn't say bra.

Where's the buggy better boys
and did you know I didn't eat
I rode the trainway coming home
despite the running films were late
when wearing reels would make me tired
and ice cream only cost a dime?

You were such a handful to
watch when I would distract you
with talkies and snacks for an
afternoon so Grandpa could
have some time off. It's taken
me eighteen years to tell you
goodbye. You can go home now.

51

God Bless You

she said, my nose skidding towards my chin.
God bless you she said again.
I tend to sneeze in pairs.
Dabbing the itch with a cotton hankie
I return to our conversation on vegetable steamers only
to see her eyes welling — *You sneeze*
just like your grandma she admits
grin piling on her cheeks.
Allergens abound and she blesses the next
with *Hello Mother*. Then we wait
without looking like we're waiting
for another sneeze.

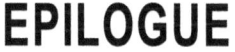

EPILOGUE

Profit From Loss

One hundred years after Watson and Crick
fifteen million will be stricken
costing seven hundred billion,
nearly double the national budgets
—defense, justice, commerce, labor—
combined.

One hundred years ago
Dr. A diagnosed Auguste D
—*nine years caught in weedy strands*—
one more year than the coming average.
Her stroke woke the giant
when autopsy gave a label: Alzheimer's.

One hundred trillion pathways
—breathing, touch, mobility, speech, arousal—
peppered with one hundred billion nerve cells
(What is the sound of one neuron lapsing?)
three pounds of power unparalleled, bewildering,
and filament fragile.

One hundred million to be freed
by the pharmaceutical dream vaccine
—heroes Salk and Sabin saved only one to two from polio—
the new market plots science on a by-line.
One-third are financially staked
publishing what pays
withholding what could save until published.
Property rights stall progress for the bottom line:
wealth innumerable.

Alzheimer's: The Cast

Bachelor
the center of his universe
lusty techno addict
seeks gyration & stimulating conversation
axons and dendrites daily
faster than fed-ex
hoping his pappy will find him
before he gets lonely
Neuron

. . .

Matchmaker
lives in 203 sprinkling
fairy dust and a prayer
may the bachelor in 204
meet someone new in 202
hosts a dinner
lighting candles and conversation
tomorrow they wed
Synapse

. . .

Valedictorian
voted most likely to be queen
mood swings wider than
her gleaming smile
can out-bench the boys
majored in ESP
limbic limbo celebrity
scrapbooking and building bunkers
her idea of a good time
Hippocampus

...

Mother hen
panic attack to go please
worry flurry scurry
wears almond-sized helmet
should the sky split wide
neighbor to limbic genius
anxious her ESP will expire
delivers a free-range organic casserole
frets she didn't prick the foil
Amygdala

...

Operator
gray her favorite color
stretched thin over no vacation days
electro-nerve surge
illumines board of callers
how may I direct your impulse?
research? admin? PR?
Hold for one planck please.
lobes of productivity
waffled oligarchy
she connecting networks
slave to the elite
Cerebral Cortex

...

Black Sheep
sleeps with only one eye shut
trigger-pappy
whadjusayernamewas?
waits for stars to align
for moonshine and nostalgia
watchtower ready
keeps every letter ever opened
but only shows them with secret handshake
knows a mountain of trails
like they lead to gold
Engram

...

Postman
blame, barred teeth, ingrown toenail
cannot stop his mail detail
sister snips shorts too short
the last stamp
goes Jekyll postal
bakes fruitcake of junk mail
winging crusty clumpy brown onto bachelor ledges
clogs limbic limbo
wedges it in windows
deeper than brush can clean
attack for eternity
Plaque

...

Sister
committed to Truth
looses The Way, brother ignores calls
faith buckles
message abandoned
bad habit seeks preymate
tapeworm thong & parasite pasties
makes a date
brings black stringy bundles
nixes dinner and candles
escape latch jammed by clumpy brown
strangles unsuspecting bachelor
Tangles

ACKNOWLEDGEMENTS

It would be most appropriate to first honor Betty McClure Nicholas, my grandmother, for living in a way that inspired those around her to live better.

I am also grateful to *Nimrod: International Journal of Prose and Poetry* for publishing *Add-a-pearl Necklace* at a crucial time in the completion of this book.

Thank you to David Shenk for his work on *The Forgetting* that was an impetus in knotting off my own. In addition, thanks to Dr. David Kellogg for encouraging this project in its infancy and for laughing at the parts that were supposed to be funny.

All perspective on this disease would be lost were it not for the staff at the Antelope Valley Nursing Center and other Alzheimer's homes that help victims and their families find dignity in the forgetting. Thank you for your tireless service.

To Laure-Anne Bosselaar, Mary Cornish, Stuart Dischell, Stephen Dobyns, Ron Egatz, Liz Irmiter, Tom Lux, James Manlow, Dean Parkin, Michael Salcman, Ellen Bryant Voigt, Dean Young and all of the other SLC poets, your support has been invaluable — next Spinning Wheel, my treat.

To my grandparents, natural and honorary, your love for family gave me the heart to write in this mad, mad world. To my parents, thank you for your love and your legacy. To Clark, Nick, Allie, Kelly, and Autumn— we have so many memories to laugh back on, and I look forward to making more with you. To my children, Josiah, Isaiah, and Evelyn, as you grow and learn to read the world I hope you will carry with you our heritage of love.

To my dear and loving husband, Josh, thank you for cherishing me in and out of season and for supporting me in countless ways so I could pursue my best work. I pray our someday passing is easier: in each other's arms, at the age of 98, smiling in our sleep after a full day scuba diving.

Praise be to God who comforts us in our mourning and turns it to laughter.

A BRIEF LOOK AT THE BIOLOGY OF ALZHEIMER'S

My great concern in writing this section is two-fold: I am neither a doctor, nor, once printed, can a book stay current with scientific advancements. However, given the complexity of Alzheimer's and my desire to make it a bit more transparent, I'm willing to risk it. (I am very grateful to Dr. Michael Salcman—neurosurgeon, poet, and friend—for honing the accuracy of this section.)

As of late, scientists can not yet agree on what causes Alzheimer's disease. They can only agree on its effect: what were once healthy, functioning parts of a brain have now been corrupted. What follows is a layman's summary of a few major parts of the brain, what they do, and how they are affected by Alzheimer's Disease.

The most basic element of the brain is the **Neuron**. A neuron's job is to pass information over synapses to other neurons at lightning speed. Like a bridge over the Grand Canyon, a **Synapse** lives in the gap between two neurons trying to communicate. To help those neurons share information, each synapse releases a chemical (a neurotransmitter) that anchors the bridge to the wall, helping impulses leap the gap from one neuron to the next.

These neurons and synapses are spread throughout the brain, but the first place they are under attack by Alzheimer's is in the **Cerebral Cortex**. An extremely complex structure, the cerebral cortex supervises the "higher functions" of life such as judgment, personality, and concentration. Part of its job is to translate sensations between four main lobes which monitor intellect, memory, communication, and input from the nervous system, to name a few.

Once the cerebral cortex has been affected, the disease moves on to the **Hippocampus**. Named for a seahorse because of its shape, the hippocampus is small but mighty, balancing a limbic system of instinct, caution, moods, and memory patterns. When it comes time to make a memory, the hippocampus collects as much data as possible before passing it along to the cerebral cortex for long-term storage.

Beside the hippocampus is the **Amygdala**, a structure small enough to be termed "the almond" by the Greeks. A minor stimulus to the amygdala can produce a physical sensation of fear on varying levels. Unfortunately, its connections to the cortex are asymmetrical, which means that it becomes increasingly harder to find the off switch once the fear has begun to flow.

Each of these parts of the brain (among others) become infected in some way by Alzheimer's via plaques or tangles, or a combination of the two. **Plaque** is a good protein (an amyloid precursor protein, to be exact) gone bad. For some reason, an enzyme got in there and snipped an otherwise healthy protein into little pieces; and, instead of being flushed away, those pieces turned sticky and balled up into a clumpy mess collecting other cell debris until the brain was littered with more sticky little clumps than the floor of a movie theatre after a busy weekend.

What made the enzyme start snipping? That's what scientists are trying to figure out. Unfortunately, as plaque grows it crowds neurons and gradually immobilizes the hippocampus, making it increasingly harder to maintain mental stability and lay down new memories (such as how to work the new cell phone). It's no wonder that when all is not right in the head, the amygdala then fires up with a growing dose of fear that becomes harder and harder to disable. It is not unusual for Alzheimer's patients to wander in a constant state of worry, as a result.

Where **Tangles** come into play is in suffocating neurons and crowding out synapses. To be fair, tangles weren't originally a disease either. Another story of protein gone bad, they originally worked within neurons (as a tau protein) to help transfer information and nutrients down a long track of microtubules. While scientists are still trying to determine the catalyst which corrupted the tau protein, what they do know is that once the protein ceases to work as it should the railway system of information collapses into a tumbleweed of knots that eventually suffocate each neuron until it dies. In autopsies, examiners have found numerous "ghost towns" of tangles where neurons once stood.

While the neurons are dying, the synapses are stranded, the cortex is clogged, the hippocampus is shrunken, and the amygdala is running amuck, the **Engrams** become irrelevant. A controversial element of memory recall (controversial in that scientists disagree with psychologists as to whether or not they actually exist) engrams are specific patterns of neurons that, when triggered, revisit a certain memory — much like pressing a specific set of keys on a flute produces one note. However, in the case of an Alzheimer's patient, even if her brain could recall which "keys" to activate there would be fewer and fewer keys (or neurons) left to play.

In short, what makes Alzheimer's so debilitating is its ability to corrupt multiple centers in the brain at once.

DIAGNOSIS AND PROGRESSION

Suffice to say, Alzheimer's Disease is difficult to diagnose. More than just forgetting details, it is an inability to process or retrieve information in response to the environment. Though a person might think he has the disease simply because he can't find his car keys, the suggestion of AD is not as much forgetting the location of the keys as it is forgetting how to use them.

Though AD cannot be formally diagnosed without a brain autopsy, doctors have created a psychiatric exam that (coupled with interviews from caregivers and a battery of other tests) can give them about 90 percent certainty as to whether or not someone has Alzheimer's. The Mini Mental State Examination is one such test frequently used to ascertain a patient's mental health in terms of AD, and its questions follow below.

What is today's date?
What day of the week is it?
What is the season?
What state are we in?
What city are we in?
What neighborhood are we in?
What building are we in?
What floor are we on?
I'm going to name three objects and I want you to repeat them back to me: street, banana, hammer.
I'd like you to count backwards from one hundred by seven. [Stop after five answers].
Can you repeat back to me the three objects I mentioned a moment ago?
[Points to any object in the room.] What do we call this?
[Points to another object.] What do we call this?
Repeat after me: "No if's, and's, or but's."

Take this piece of paper in your right hand, fold it in half, and put it on the floor.

[Without speaking, doctor shows the patient a piece of paper with "Close your eyes" printed on it.]

Please write a sentence for me. It can say anything at all, but make it a complete sentence.

Here is a diagram of two intersecting pentagons. Please copy this drawing onto a plain piece of paper.

Depending on caregiver help, prior mental health, age, and physical well being, once a patient has been diagnosed with AD it can last anywhere from two to twenty years. Each patient's progression through AD is unique in its timing, though many tend to advance through the disease as outlined by Dr. Barry Reisberg's Functional Assessment Staging (FAST) scale.

STAGE ONE

No cognitive decline. No subjective complaints of memory deficit. No memory deficit evident on clinical interviews.

STAGE TWO (FORGETFULNESS)

Very mild cognitive decline. Subjective complaints of memory deficit, most frequently in forgetting where he has placed familiar objects or forgetting names he formerly knew well. No objective evidence of memory deficit on clinical interview. No objective deficits in employment or social situations. Appropriate concern regarding symptoms.

STAGE THREE (EARLY CONFUSIONAL)

Mild cognitive decline. Manifestations in more than one of the following areas: patient may have gotten lost when traveling to an unfamiliar location; coworkers become aware of patient's relatively low performance; word and name finding deficit becomes evident to intimates; patient may read a passage of a book and retain relatively little material; patient may demonstrate decreased ability to remember names upon introduction to new people; patient may have lost or misplaced an object of value; concentration deficit may be evident on clinical testing. Objective evidence of memory deficit obtained only with an intensive interview. Patient begins to manifest denial as well as mild to moderate anxiety.

STAGE FOUR (LATE CONFUSIONAL)
Moderate cognitive decline evident in clinical interview. Deficit manifests in the following areas: decreased knowledge of current and recent events; may exhibit some lack of memory concerning his personal history; decreased ability to travel or handle finances, inability to perform complex tasks. Denial is the dominant defense mechanism.

STAGE FIVE (EARLY DEMENTIA)
Moderately severe cognitive decline. Patient can no longer survive without some assistance. Patient is unable during interview to recall a major relevant aspect of his current life, such as an address or telephone number, the names of grandchildren, the name of the high school or college from which he graduated. Frequently some disorientation regarding time or place. Invariably knows his own name and generally knows his spouse's and children's names. Requires no assistance with toileting and eating, but may have some difficulty choosing the proper clothing to wear.

STAGE SIX (MIDDLE DEMENTIA)

Severe cognitive decline. May occasionally forget the name of his spouse. Will be largely unaware of recent events and surroundings. May retain some knowledge of his past life. May have difficulty counting from 10, both backward and sometimes forward. Personality and emotional changes occur and may include: delusional behavior, obsessive symptoms, anxiety agitation, suspicion. Will require some assistance with activities of daily living. Frequently continues to be able to distinguish familiar from unfamiliar persons in his environment. Can almost always recall his own name.

STAGE SEVEN (LATE DEMENTIA)

Very severe cognitive decline. All verbal abilities are lost. Frequently there is no speech at all - only grunting. Requires assistance toileting and feeding. Has lost basic psychomotor skills. The brain appears to no longer be able to tell the body what to do.

BEHIND THE POEMS

I love poetry. I love its music. I love how, in a few short lines, a poem can establish scene, character, and insight, and then wrap up just as quickly as it began in a tidy little self-sustained package. But. Sometimes I wish there was a little more— something a bit more personable beyond the poem itself.

Yes, I know. How silly of me to miss the off-the-cuff banter a poet gives right before her reading when I am merely sitting alone in my living room with her book in my hands. It's just that I think the whole experience would be a lot more fun if I had some company.

Please don't misunderstand. I'm not suggesting that poets include any sort of summary or analysis beside their poems, more something along the lines of a tour guide saying, *We are about to enter the foyer and, while you admire its artistry and exquisite structure, be sure to look for the gargoyle hidden in the upper left corner that has the face of the bishop's wife.* You know, a few random facts that acknowledge the life behind the art.

In the event you, dear reader, feel the same I have included a series of remarks to point out gargoyles and Dymo marker tape simply for your pleasure. However, to keep things sporting, this collection is at the back of the book.

Best of reading to you.
Anne

Add-a-pearl Necklace

This is actually the first and only Alzheimer's poem I have published in a poetry journal. It wasn't for lack of trying, either. I have a sizable stack of rejection letters spanning eight years saying the poems were "good, but too focused on Alzheimer's." I kind of thought that was the point. *Nimrod* asked to include this poem in their edition on memory, and I am grateful.

The Mini Mental State Examination for Alzheimer's in Recitative

This poem is based off the actual questions used to test a patient's mental acuity. Don't be surprised if you find yourself answering them part way through (and don't be too rough on yourself if you can't remember the three objects.) The actual test questions are listed in the Appendix, and it is one of many tests used to diagnose Alzheimer's disease.

Old-Timers

Apart from their off-handed references to "Old-timers," I don't recall my grandparents discussing Alzheimer's much. Individually, they spoke with us about the disease on occasion but it seems to have been a subject they didn't speak about to one another much at all, at least not publicly. I'm sure it heightened for them what was already a lonely disease.

Stage Three

I used an unraveling form of the sestina for this poem because the obsessive nature of worry seemed to pair well with the repetition of line endings. Even though the end words morph into homonyms as her speech deteriorates, her worry remains constant. (For those who are new to the sestina form, the same six words must be used to end six stanzas of six lines each in the specific pattern that is used here.)

Aria of the Caretaker

When I was little, Grandma used to read me a book called *This is the House that Jack Built* where each line built on the one previous until the final page had an enormous laundry list of things Jack built one after another. It must have been a torturous book for an adult to read aloud over and over, but as a child I loved it. Originally, I thought to mimic the pattern purely for sentimental reasons, but as the poem got going, I liked how the pattern lent itself to obsession naturally. Of course, by the end I wonder what business the patient even has driving a car!

Above the Unraveling

As a former accountant, Grandpa was best friends with his Dymo-marker gun. Some of my earliest memories are of him stamping out the proper locations for a box of golf tees, various keys, and, of course, where the gun itself was to be stored. After Grandpa died and we began clearing out his apartment, my uncle gasped when he pulled open the sock drawer—inside lay rows of neatly folded socks arranged in order of ascending color. Even now I'm frightened to admit how much this level of organization appeals to me, and as a result have never asked for a labeling gun for Christmas.

Belaboring Dead Horses

It took me nearly eight years to write this poem, largely because when I conceived the idea my skills weren't up to the challenge of writing a double sestina (a form where words repeat according to a set pattern both on the ends as well as within the lines). If the insanity of the patient doesn't show in the poem, perhaps the insanity of the poet does.

Stage Five

Butter Pecan was Grandma's favorite flavor of ice cream. If ever there was a time I visited her house and there wasn't a half-gallon in the freezer, she considered it a major oversight and would find some excuse to drive to the grocery that afternoon. Even after she forgot most everything else, when we took her on outings to Baskin-Robbins that's what she would order. It wasn't until the end of her illness, when we moved her into an Alzheimer's ward and she no longer had access to a freezer, that she lost those butter pecan pounds and I saw her face appear, like her old black and white photos, for the first time.

Waltz

Grandpa was so tickled the day he got the idea of buying a "boom box" from the drugstore to play background music for Grandma on one of his visits to the ward. It was a surprise to both he and the nurses when she started dancing along with the music, and he brought the boom box every week after that. Sometimes she was up for a dance and many times she wasn't. What I admired about him so much was that he drove nearly two hours each way, three times a week, to visit her regardless. The nurses absolutely loved him.

Caregiver Support Group: First Meeting This Thursday

I've never understood why so many of my grandparents' lifetime friends disappeared once Grandma was diagnosed with Alzheimer's, especially after they had already survived so much together. I imagine their pause was largely motivated by ignorance. One of my goals with this collection is to show how Alzheimer's progresses and how loved ones play an important role despite the forgetting.

Conundrum

This poem is, to me, the heartbeat of this collection. Its nagging question is what drove me to write and wouldn't let me rest until the book was published. Writing these poems for nearly twenty years has been my way of saying goodbye.

Photo Caption: Betty recites the 23rd Psalm

After Grandma was moved to the ward, Grandpa would regularly mail us photos from their visits so we could see her new room, her scowl as she modeled a sweatshirt we sent, or how the flowers were blooming outside her window. Nearly all of the photos were of Grandma sitting alone staring at the camera with an unnerving expression of suspicion or vacancy. It was almost like looking at a picture of a picture. Despite her demeanor, Grandpa would write something positive on the back of the photo that had happened during his visit, and the irony of this particular caption made it one of my favorites.

The Real Question

What is it like to lose someone to Alzheimer's — to evolve from that state of beloved to stranger? For my younger brothers who don't really have memories of Grandma prior to the onset of her disease, they are a little perplexed why I have been so consumed with the subject. Even trying to share this burden with my husband — how Grandma's final darkness over-shadows all my happy memories of her — seems incomplete. How does a soul explain what it feels like to have the wind knocked out of it? Worse yet, what do we do with the nagging terror of which one of us may be next?

Nurses Thought We Should Know

This was one of those conversations we had with Grandma in the later stages that exemplifies how Alzheimer's abused her most private memories. Prior to this disease — even after nearly fifty years of marriage — she had never told her husband that she had been molested as a child. And, she probably wouldn't have. She had told her daughters, however, and it was their unfortunate task to confirm to him what she was saying after she had been admitted to the ward.

Riding Dead Horses

There were certain memories that Grandma seemed to relive daily, even long after she didn't know our faces or names. To me, that seemed the most torturous part of the disease — not just that she would forget her loved ones but that she would dwell on the memories she would have chosen to forget first, and that she would have to endure them alone.

It's Only Money

Oh, don't worry — to some extent we all think we have It.

Unscrambling Her Forgetting

I guarantee I won't be reading this anagram publicly.

Condolences

There came a point in the grieving process when the silver linings and best wishes and loving sentiments all seemed to blur into a blob of color that sometimes brightened a dark moment but other times felt like a mush of words. Since the latter was the stronger for me, I used this prose poem form — which I typically don't enjoy — to give that run-on effect those best wishes had for me.

End Stage

Some therapists theorize that at the end of Alzheimer's — when there is very little left of memory or physical function — the patient can finally reach a state of living rest, almost floating above the cares that keep the rest of us running in our hamster wheels. One can only hope they're right.

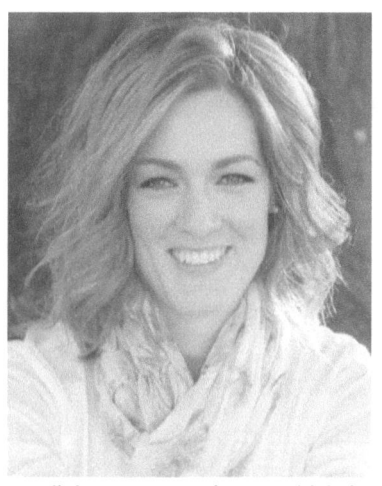

Author, poet, and educator, **Anne Crossman** made her publishing debut with *Getting the Best Out of College: A Professor, a Dean, and a Student Tell You How to Maximize Your Experience* (Ten Speed Press, 2008).

After studying at Stanford and Duke Universities, Anne taught in public high schools, military barracks, and around kitchen tables to students ranging from academic underdogs to honor society prodigies, an experience which inspired her third book, *Study Smart, Study Less* (Ten Speed Press, 2011).

Her work has been published in notable sources such as the *Washington Post*, *Margie*, and *Nimrod*. *Trying to Remember* is her first book of poems.

www.AnneCrossman.com